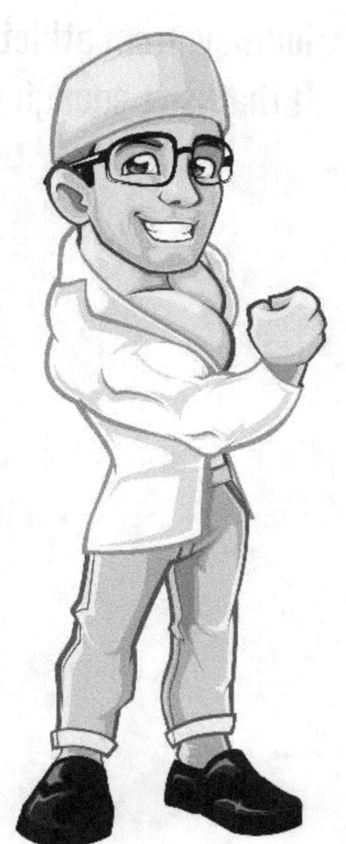

I0693403

Introduction: Why Should You Listen to Me?

Who am I, and why should you listen to me ramble about health, fitness, and wellness for the next few chapters? Well, let's just say I'm not your average health guru spouting out generic advice like, "Eat less, move more." My name is Dr. Victor Prisk, and I've worn many hats in my life: orthopedic surgeon, professional bodybuilder, nutrition expert, and even a guy who's had to fix his fair share of broken bones—both figuratively and literally. My journey, from athlete to surgeon, is a unique one that I hope will inspire and intrigue you. If that isn't enough to earn your attention, let's hope my jokes keep you around.

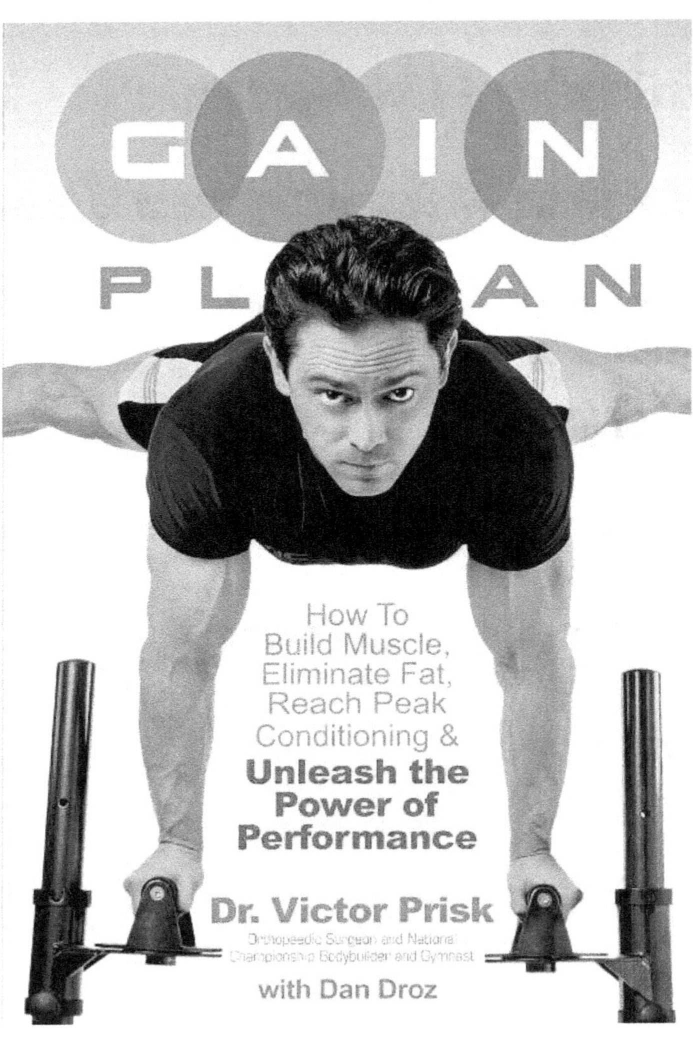

Let's start with why I wrote this book. I deeply love helping people achieve their health goals, especially when they've been told their best days are behind them. In my career as an orthopedic surgeon, I've seen the impact that injuries, bad health habits, and sometimes just plain bad luck can have on a person. But I've also seen the incredible power of what happens when someone takes control of their body and mind, using the right tools to get stronger, healthier, and happier. This love for helping people is at the heart of this book, and I hope it makes you feel cared for and understood. I realized that my approach with my patients could help anyone—whether they were recovering from an injury, trying to lose weight, or just wanting to live their best life without feeling like they needed a nap every afternoon.

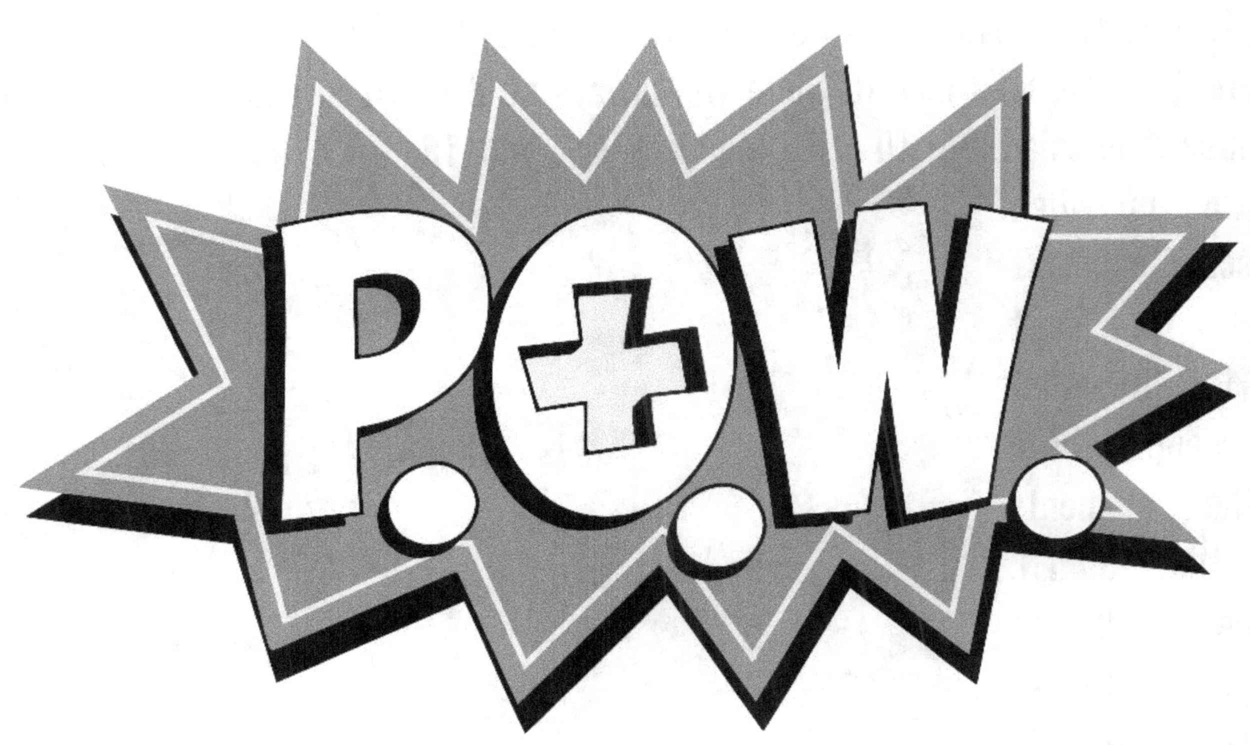

The G.A.I.N. Plan is my answer to that need. It's built around four principles that have stood the test of time—Graded Exercise, Attitude, Integrated Medicine, and Nutrition. Each of these pillars plays a crucial role in creating a sustainable, well-rounded, healthy lifestyle. You don't need a perfect body or superhuman willpower to get started. All you need is a willingness to take the first step—and maybe a sense of humor to laugh through the stumbles. Trust me, there will be stumbles.

If you're anything like my patients, you might feel a little overwhelmed. You may have tried countless diets, workout regimens, and health trends that promised miracles and delivered disappointment. You might feel like your body is betraying you, that no matter what you do, you can't seem to get the results you want. Well, I'm here to tell you it's not about finding the perfect, one-size-fits-all solution. It's about understanding your body, fueling it properly, moving in a way that works for you, and developing the mindset to persevere. Because let's face it, there will always be days when pizza just seems like a better idea than salad. But I'll also be honest with you. There will be days when you feel like giving up when the scale doesn't budge, or you can't seem to lift that heavier weight. These are the moments when the G.A.I.N. principles will be tested, but they're also the moments when you'll see the most growth.

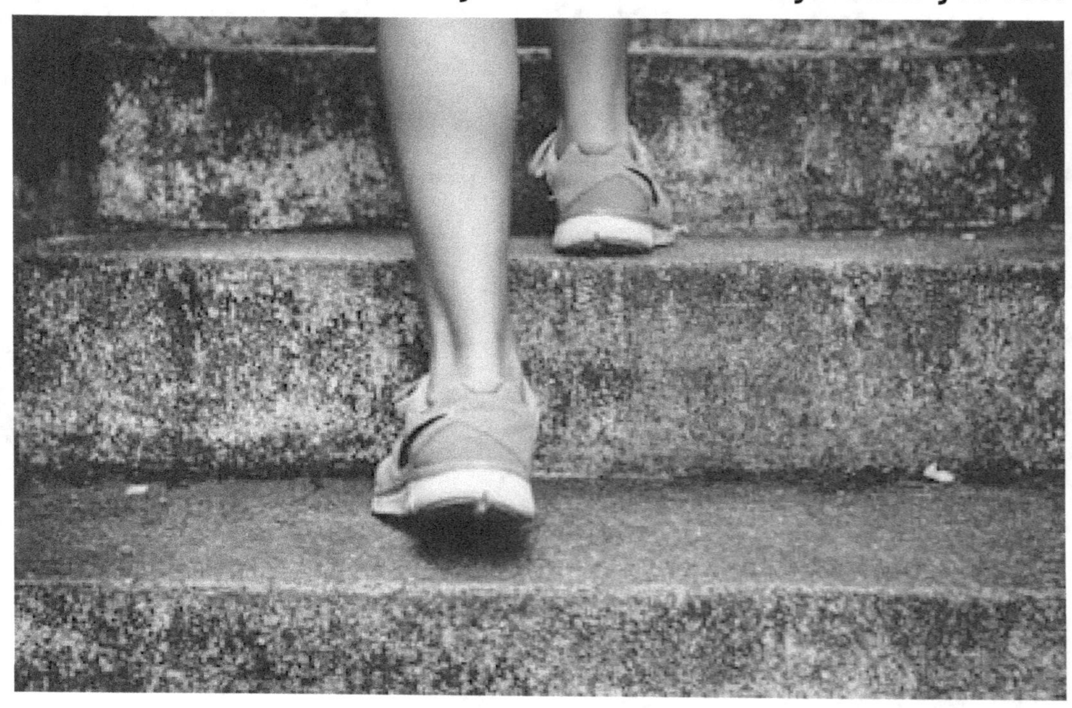

Now, let's talk a bit about my journey. I didn't wake up one day and decide, "Hey, I think I'll be a doctor who also knows a thing or two about lifting weights." My journey to becoming a health and wellness guide was a long and sometimes painful one. I started my career as an athlete—a gymnast, to be precise. That led me to bodybuilding, where I learned the ins and outs of nutrition, exercise, and the sheer willpower it takes to get back up every time you fall (or every time you drop a barbell on your foot). Eventually, I became an orthopedic surgeon, where I started applying what I learned about training and nutrition to my patients. I realized that whether you're an elite athlete or someone who's never set foot in a gym, the principles of G.A.I.N. can change your life if you're willing to work for it. This book is the culmination of my experiences, the lessons I've learned, and the strategies that have proven effective for me and my patients.

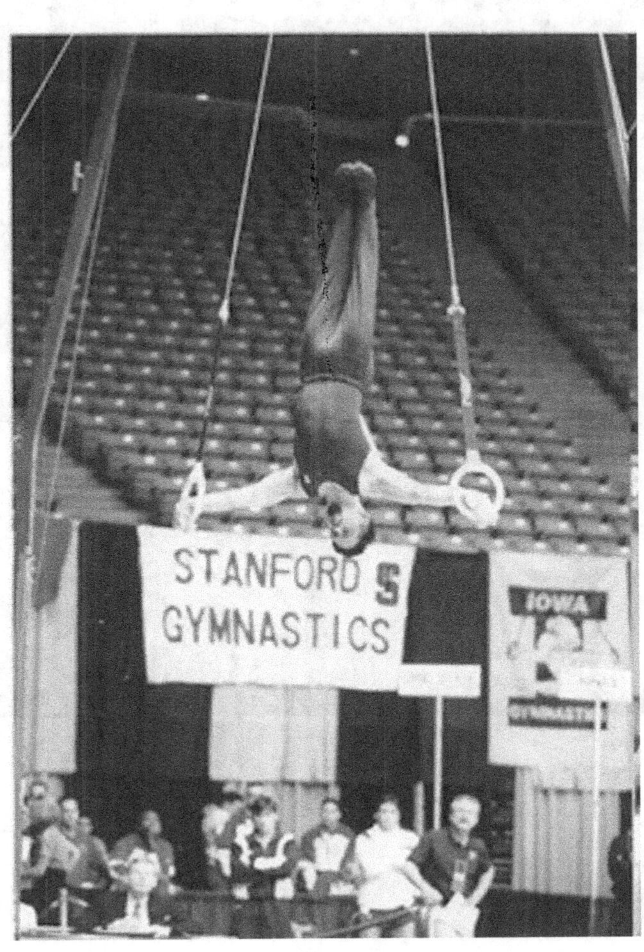

This book is going to take you on a journey through the G.A.I.N. principles: Graded Exercise, Attitude, Integrated Medicine, and Nutrition. I'm not promising it will be easy, but I can promise it will be worth it. We're going to cover a lot of ground—everything from how to move in a way that helps you get stronger without breaking down, to why leucine is your new best friend when it comes to building muscle (hint: it's not a magical potion, but it's pretty close). We'll talk about what it takes to adjust your attitude, use integrative approaches to health, and make nutrition work for you, not against you. And yes, I'll try to make you laugh a little along the way—because let's face it, health can be a pretty serious topic, but that doesn't mean we have to take ourselves too seriously. I want you to feel hopeful and optimistic about the journey ahead.

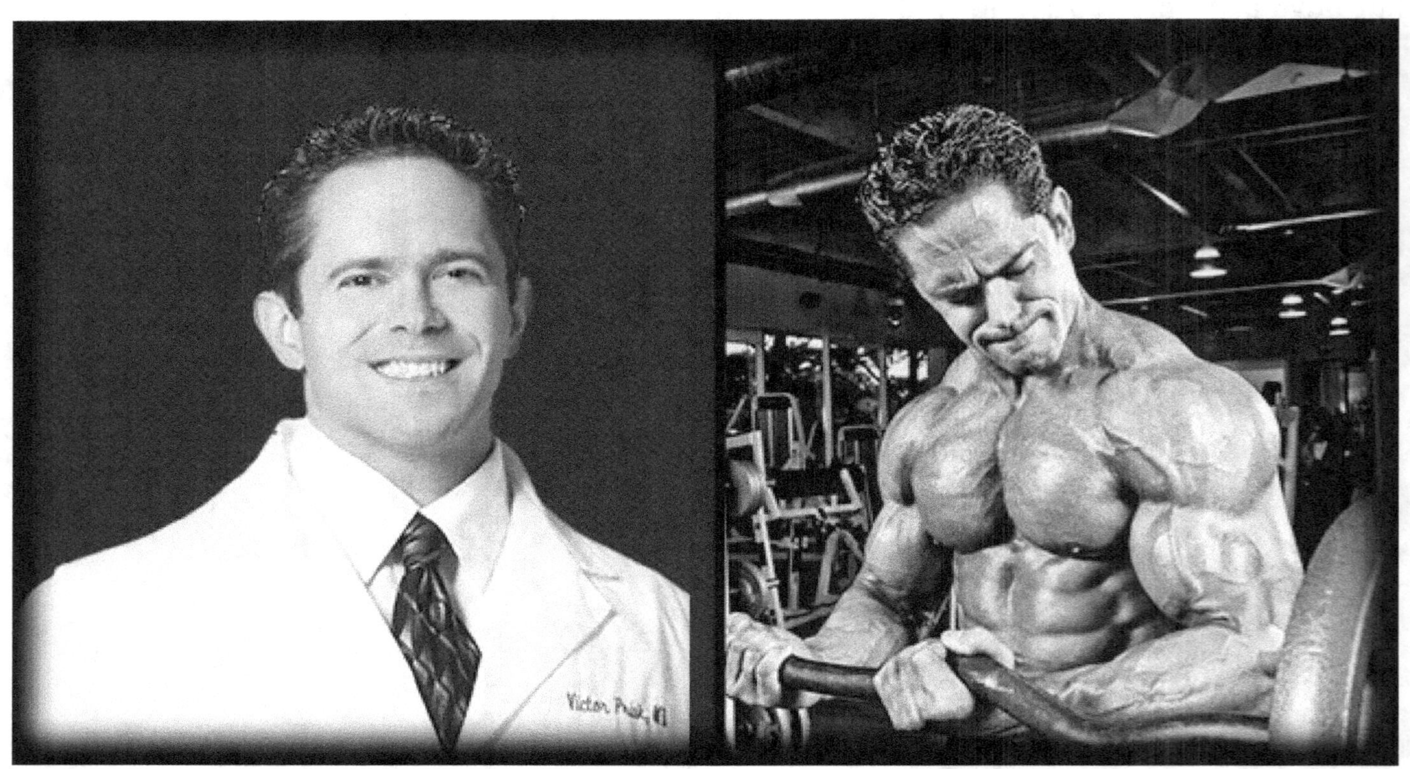

If at any point you're wondering whether all of this is possible for you, remember this: I've seen patients who could barely walk make incredible strides (literally and figuratively), and I've seen regular people do extraordinary things with just a little guidance and a lot of determination. My goal is to be that guide for you—to show you that you're capable of far more than you realize and to give you the tools to take control of your health and write a better story for yourself.

So, let's dive in. This isn't just another health book; it's a guide to getting your life back on track in a way that works for you—without the stress, without the gimmicks, and maybe even with a few laughs. Let's G.A.I.N. your health back, one step at a time. And remember: laughter is a core exercise, so get those abs ready.

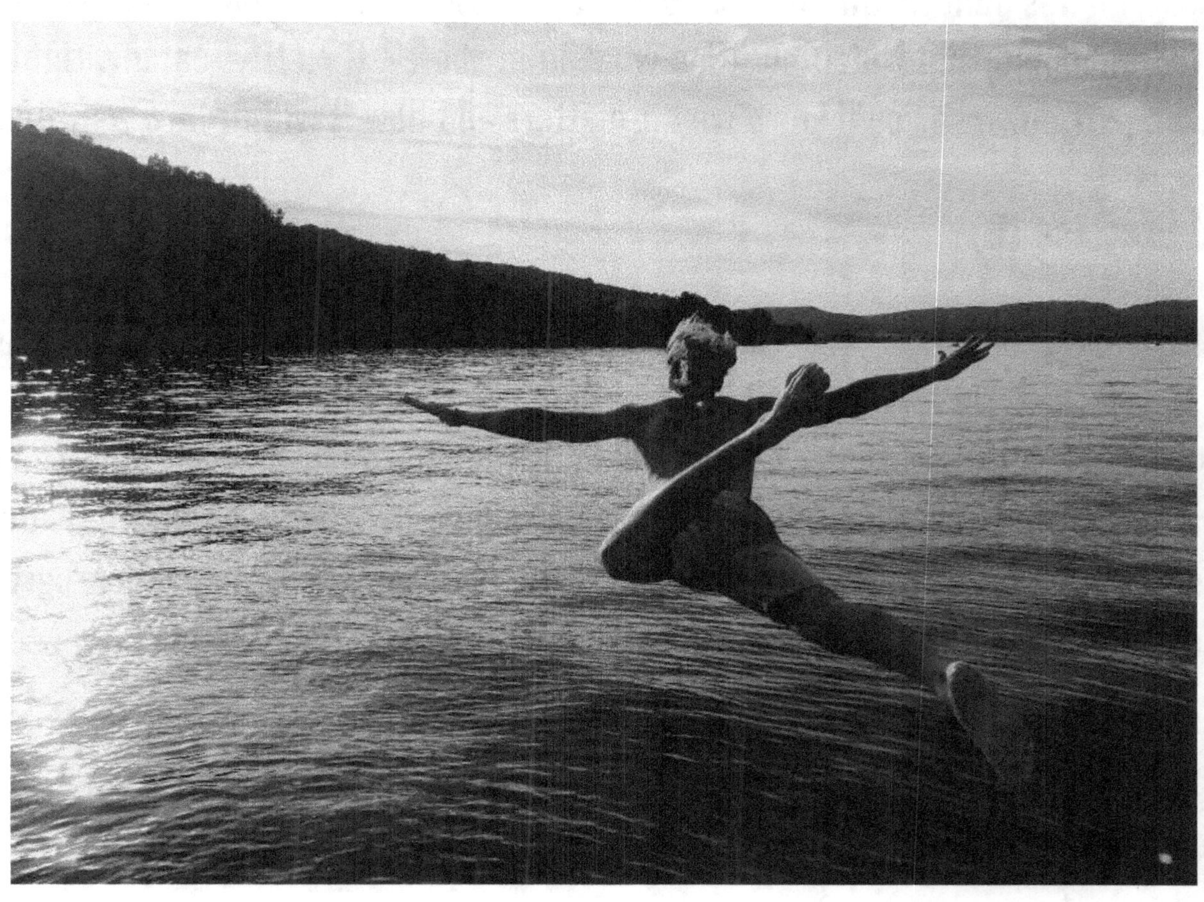

Chapter 1: The G.A.I.N. Formula—A Roadmap to Wellness

Fuel Your Mind, Strengthen Your Body

Welcome to the G.A.I.N. Formula, your personalized roadmap to feeling and moving better. If you've ever wondered why all those trendy health plans seem to work for everyone but you, they often focus on just one piece of the puzzle. The G.A.I.N. Plan is different—it's a four-part powerhouse designed to address every aspect of your wellness, from what you eat to how you think. And don't worry, I promise not to turn you into a science experiment... unless, of course, you're into that sort of thing.

The G.A.I.N. Plan is built around four simple yet powerful pillars: Graded Exercise, Attitude, Integrated Medicine, and Nutrition. (See what I did there? G.A.I.N.—catchy, right?) Let's break each part down so you'll know why it matters and how it will fit into your life.

Graded Exercise (G)

Think of Graded Exercise as your "Goldilocks" approach to working out—not too much, not too little, but just right. It's all about starting at the appropriate level and gradually turning up the heat, like that slow cooker chili that gets better over time (minus the potential heartburn). Whether you're looking to bounce back from an injury or get those muscles popping for beach season, graded exercise is the key to sustainable progress—no overdoing it until you can't get off the couch the next day.

If you're envisioning hours of torture on a treadmill, rest easy. This isn't about marathon sessions or becoming a bodybuilder overnight (trust me, I've been there—it's a lot of protein shakes). Instead, Graded Exercise is tailored to help you make slow and steady gains that add up over time. After all, Rome wasn't built in a day, and neither are quads of steel.

Attitude (A)

Let's talk about that thing between your ears—no, not your AirPods. Your attitude is a powerful part of your wellness journey. It's not about having a Tony Robbins motivational poster on your wall (though, if it works, go for it). It's about cultivating a mindset that lets you keep pushing forward, even when life throws in a few extra speed bumps—like holiday dinners with those relatives who insist on deep-fried everything.

This chapter will help you understand how your mindset shapes your health and success. We'll discuss practical exercises to keep you mentally strong, and yes, some positive self-talk may be involved. If talking to yourself isn't your thing, pretend you're rehearsing for your Oscar speech—you know, for Best Attitude in a Leading Role.

Integrated Medicine (I)

Next, we've got Integrated Medicine. This might sound like a buzzword for people who collect crystals (and hey, no judgment if you do). Still, integrated medicine combines the best of mainstream medical science with complementary therapies. It's like the best of both worlds, without needing to chant under a full moon. From physical therapy to joint health supplements, these strategies help you recover better, prevent injuries, and get back to doing what you love—whether that's hitting the gym or simply tying your shoes without feeling like you've run a marathon.

Imagine having a whole toolkit at your disposal, not just a hammer. We'll cover how these tools can work together to support your health. After all, if Thor can carry around a whole bunch of magical tools, so can you (just fewer lightning bolts involved).

Nutrition (N)

Finally, there's Nutrition—the fuel that keeps everything else running smoothly. But we're not talking about boring salads and kale smoothies here (unless, of course, you love kale, in which case... I'm sorry). Nutrition is about getting the proper nutrients at the right time to support your body and mind. The star of the show is leucine, a superstar amino acid that helps build muscle and keep you energized. It's kind of like the secret sauce that makes all those other nutrients work harder, which means you get better results without living on celery sticks.

We'll delve into the power of leucine and how to incorporate it into your meals in a practical, non-lab-experiment way. You'll be pleasantly surprised at how delicious and satisfying healthy food can be when it's working for you, not against you.

Pulling It All Together

When you combine Graded Exercise, Attitude, Integrated Medicine, and Nutrition, you create a holistic approach that's more than the sum of its parts. Each pillar is crucial on its own, but when they work together, that's when the real magic happens. And by magic, I mean fundamental, lasting changes that you can actually stick with—no disappearing acts required.

Throughout this book, you're going to learn how to put each of these pillars into practice, one step at a time. My goal isn't just to give you information—it's to give you a roadmap you can follow that feels manageable, even when life gets busy. There will be no "one-size-fits-all" solutions here, just a framework that you can adapt to your own needs and goals.

And if at any point you think, "Well, this sounds impossible," just remember—I've seen people do some incredible things, often starting from rock bottom. We're in this together, and as long as you're willing to put in the work, I promise you'll see the benefits.

Let's get started. After all, this is your story—I'm just here to help you write a healthier, more substantial ending.

(And yes, there will be humor along the way—laughter is good for the abs, after all.)

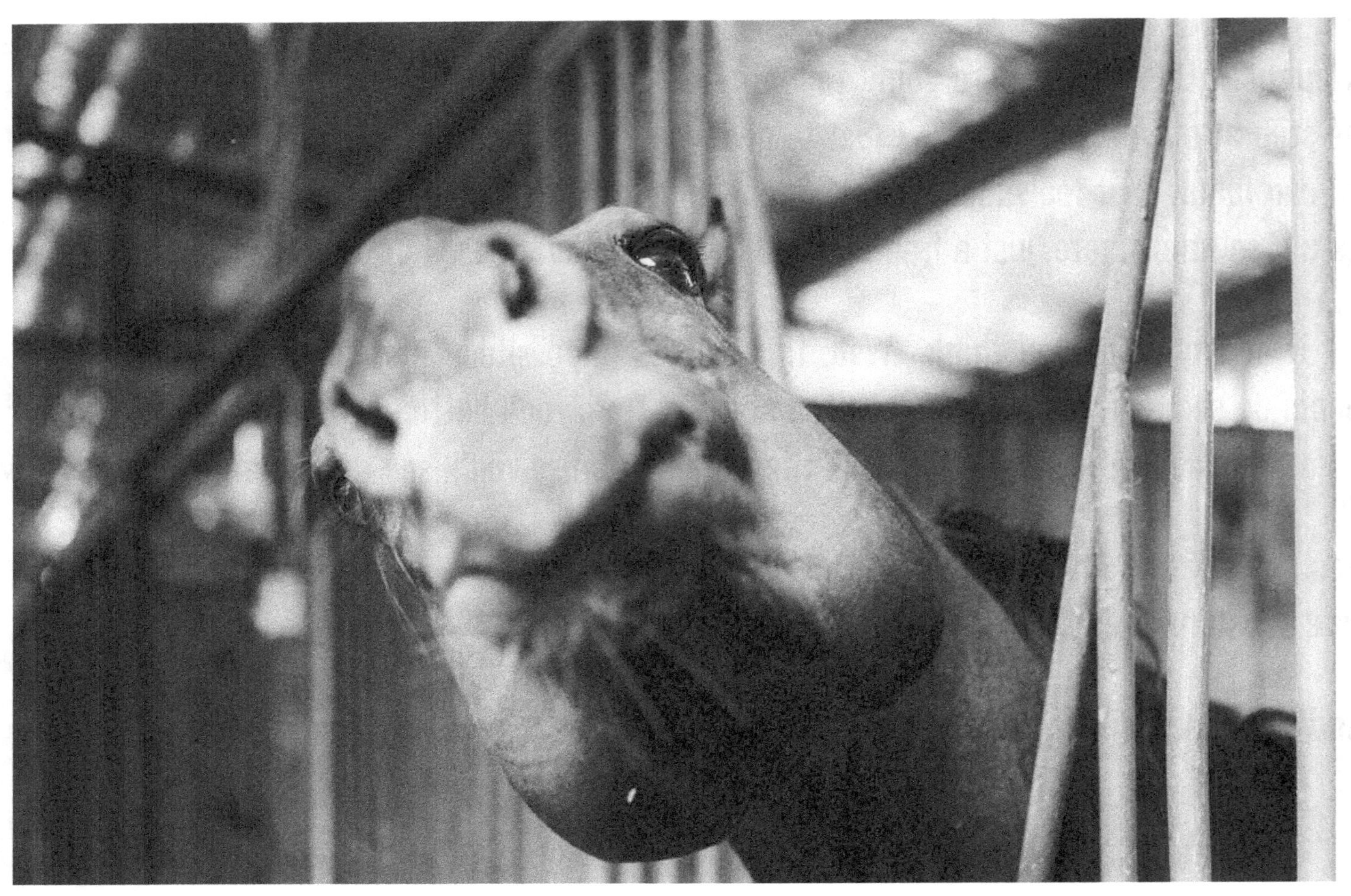

Chapter 2: Building the Foundation—The Truth About Your Body

Welcome to a world where health myths are busted, and your body's potential is finally revealed. Please think of this chapter as a friendly chat with someone who's seen the worst (trust me, broken bones can be graphic) and knows how to get you feeling your best. By debunking these myths, you'll gain a new level of confidence in your health decisions.

The Human Body: It's More Than Meets the Eye

Our bodies are complex machines, engineered for greatness but susceptible to misinformation. Let's set the record straight, debunking myths that have long overshadowed the simple truths of health. Understanding the truth about nutrition gives you a sense of control over your health and wellness.

Myth #1: Carbs Are Always the Bad Guy

We need to talk about carbs. Are they really plotting to ruin your diet? Yes, when we're discussing sugar-laden, refined carbs masquerading as healthy options. Smoothies brimming with fruit syrups or snacks marketed as "all-natural" (like those sneaky Fruit Roll-Ups) can derail your wellness journey.

The Truth: *Complex carbohydrates—like oats, quinoa, and sweet potatoes—are your allies, providing sustained energy. But it's crucial to choose whole foods over processed impostors. Your body deserves fuel, not sugar bombs.*

Myth #2: Fat Will Make You Fat

It's time to stop fearing fat. Avocados, olive oil, and even a hearty handful of nuts belong in your diet. But trans fats? Now, that's a different story. These are the true culprits lurking in processed and fried foods.

The Truth: *Healthy fats support your hormones, brain function, and overall vitality. So, don't skip the guacamole (just maybe not the whole bowl in one sitting).*

Myth #3: Weightlifting Will Make You Bulky

Ladies, especially, hear this one: strength training won't make you look like a professional bodybuilder unless you actively work to get there (and consume an *astonishing* amount of calories). In reality, lifting weights is one of the best ways to improve bone density, boost metabolism, and prevent age-related muscle loss. Dispelling these exercise myths can bring a sense of relief and confidence to your fitness routine.

The Truth: Strength training helps you build lean muscle, which burns calories even at rest. So go ahead, pick up those weights—your future self will thank you.

Myth #4: More Exercise = Better Results

More isn't always better. *Yes, even in exercise.* Overtraining can lead to injuries, burnout, and hormone imbalances. Remember: quality trumps quantity.

The Truth: Exercise smarter, not harder. Incorporate rest days and focus on form rather than sheer volume. Your body needs recovery to grow stronger.

Myth #5: You Need to Eat Every Two Hours

We've been led to believe that constant grazing keeps our metabolism revved up. But let's debunk that one, too. Studies show that eating five to six meals a day isn't necessary for fat loss or metabolic boost. However, diets are a lifestyle, and all lifestyles have different patterns. Building muscle requires regular protein meals and 4 to 5 per day. Some schedules only allow 2 to 3 meals per day.

The Truth: Focus on balanced, nutrient-dense meals, and pay attention to your body's hunger cues. It's more about quality nutrition than strict eating schedules.

Bonus Principle: Listen to Your Body

If you take away one thing from this chapter, let it be this: Listen to your body. It's smarter than you think. If something feels wrong, it probably is. Pain, fatigue, and discomfort aren't signs of weakness; they're red flags your body is waving to get your attention.

Practical Tip: Learn to differentiate between soreness from a good workout and pain signaling an injury. Rest isn't laziness—it's a critical part of your wellness routine.

The Science of Nutrition and Muscle

This section dives deeper into what "fueling your body" truly means. Protein synthesis, the role of leucine, and the necessity of amino acids aren't just bodybuilding jargon. They're the foundation for keeping your metabolism healthy and your muscles strong.

Myth #6: High Protein Diets Will Destroy Your Kidneys

Unless you have pre-existing kidney conditions, a higher protein intake is safe for most people. In fact, protein is crucial for muscle maintenance and metabolic health.

The Truth: Eating adequate protein, especially if you're active, helps repair and build muscle tissue. Pair it with plenty of water, and you're all set.

Putting It All Together

Your body is adaptable but not invincible. Understanding these myths and principles gives you the power to make informed choices, avoid unnecessary setbacks, and build a wellness plan that works for you. The G.A.I.N. approach is about balance: eating, moving, and resting in harmony.

Remember: Health is not about extremes but sustainable, enjoyable habits. Let's debunk myths, learn what makes our bodies thrive, and—most importantly—give ourselves the grace to get there, one step at a time.

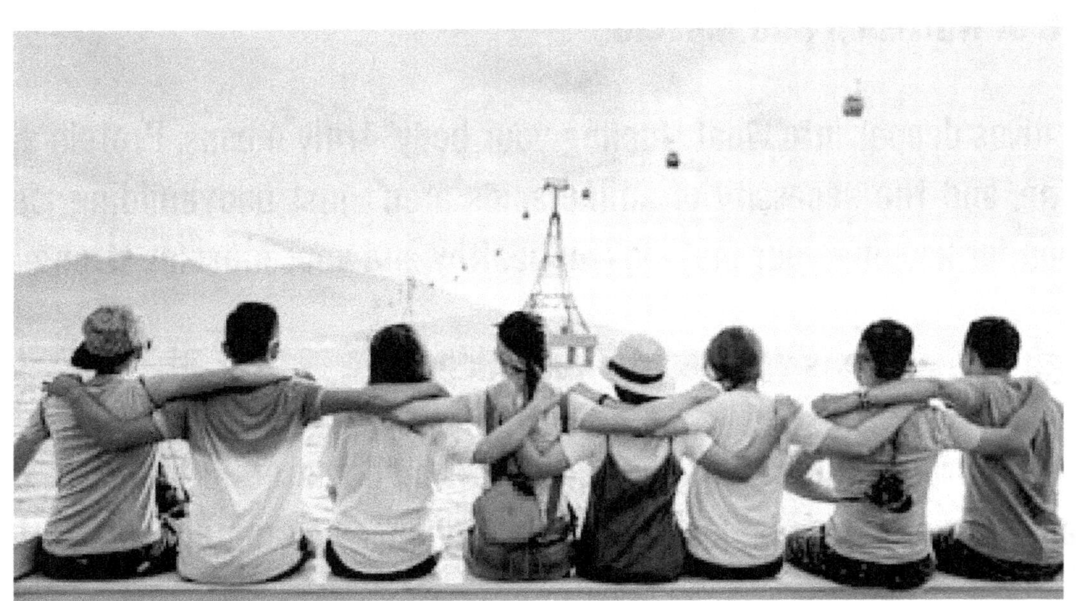

Chapter 3: Creating Your Blueprint for Lasting Health

Now that we've laid the groundwork by busting myths and giving you a fresh perspective on your body, it's time to get practical. This chapter is your personalized playbook for making real, lasting changes to your health and well-being. Think of it as your go-to guide for building the kind of healthy routines that you won't abandon faster than a New Year's resolution.

The Power of Routine

Routines are more than just habits; they're the backbone of sustainable change. Our bodies crave consistency. Whether it's the time you go to bed or your daily protein intake, having a set routine can make a world of difference.

Graded Exercise: Creating Your Movement Plan

You don't need to be a gym rat to benefit from regular exercise. In fact, one of the biggest mistakes people make is diving headfirst into grueling workouts without a plan. Here's where *Graded Exercise* comes in.

Step 1: Assess Your Starting Point

Take a moment to evaluate where you are right now. Have you been sedentary for years? Are you recovering from an injury? Or are you an athlete looking to level up? Your starting point determines your approach.

Step 2: Create a Balanced Workout Schedule

- **Strength Training:** Two to three days a week. Focus on compound movements like squats, lunges, and push-ups, which work for multiple muscle groups.
- **Cardiovascular Health:** Walking, cycling, or swimming. Start slow and work your way up.
- **Flexibility and Recovery:** Yoga, foam rolling, and rest days are essential to avoid injury.

Remember: Your workout plan should feel challenging but not impossible. The goal is to make gradual progress.

Attitude: Cultivating a Growth Mindset

A healthy body starts with a healthy mind. It's easy to get discouraged when progress feels slow, but a growth mindset can make all the difference.

Visualize Your Success

Athletes often use visualization to prepare for competitions. Picture yourself completing a workout, eating a nourishing meal, or achieving a goal. It primes your brain for success.

Celebrate Small Wins

Did you hit a new personal best at the gym? Manage to meal-prep for the week? Take time to acknowledge these victories. They're stepping stones to more significant accomplishments.

Integrated Medicine: A Holistic Approach

Your health isn't just about how many steps you took today. Integrated medicine considers the bigger picture, from stress management to injury prevention.

Physical Therapy and Preventive Care

Got a nagging pain? Don't ignore it. A visit to a physical therapist can help prevent long-term damage. Think of it as maintenance for your body, like getting an oil change for your car.

Supplements and Joint Health

This is where targeted supplementation comes in. Collagen, omega-3s, and magnesium are just a few of the supplements that support joint health and recovery.

Pro Tip: *Always consult with a healthcare provider before starting a new supplement regimen.*

Nutrition: Meal Planning for Your Goals

It's time to put the principles of *The Leucine Factor Diet* into action. Meal planning doesn't have to be a chore; it can actually be empowering.

Step 1: Build Your Leucine-Rich Plate

- **Protein:** Aim for lean meats, eggs, dairy, or plant-based options like tofu and legumes.
- **Complex Carbs:** Sweet potatoes, quinoa, or brown rice. These provide sustained energy without the blood sugar rollercoaster.
- **Healthy Fats:** Avocados, nuts, or olive oil. They help with hormone production and keep you satiated.

Step 2: Meal Timing

This doesn't mean eating every two hours but instead fueling your body when it needs it most, like post-workout. *Hint:* Aim for a protein-rich snack within 30 minutes of exercise.

Bonus: Creating a Wellness Journal

Consider keeping a wellness journal to track your workouts, meals, and how you're feeling. It's a great way to spot patterns and celebrate your progress. Plus, it's therapeutic to put pen to paper.

By the end of this chapter, you should have a clear vision of what your day-to-day health routine will look like. Remember, this blueprint is unique to you. It's about creating habits that fit your lifestyle and bring you closer to your health goals.

Ready to put this into action? Let's G.A.I.N. some momentum together!

Chapter 4: Graded Exercise—Moving with Purpose

Exercise isn't just about sweat and sore muscles. It's a powerful tool that, when used correctly, can improve your quality of life, boost your mental health, and keep you resilient against injuries. In this chapter, we'll explore how to move with intention and make fitness an integral part of your daily routine.

The Graded Approach: Start Where You Are

Before jumping into any fitness program, it's crucial to acknowledge your current physical condition. Whether you're recovering from an injury, getting back into exercise after years of inactivity, or a seasoned athlete looking to improve, the *Graded Exercise* approach meets you where you are.

Step 1: Self-Assessment

- **Mobility Check:** Can you touch your toes? How does your back feel when you bend or twist?
- **Strength Gauge:** How many push-ups or squats can you do with good form?
- **Endurance Evaluation:** How do you feel after climbing a few flights of stairs or taking a brisk walk?

Pro Tip: If you're unsure, consider consulting a physical therapist or fitness professional. Personalized assessments can highlight areas of weakness or imbalance.

Designing Your Exercise Plan

With your starting point established, let's craft a workout plan that builds strength, improves flexibility, and enhances cardiovascular health—all while minimizing the risk of injury.

Strength Training: Building Functional Muscle

Strength training isn't just for bodybuilders. It's about creating a body that can lift, carry, and move through life with ease.

Frequency: Aim for 2-3 days per week.

Fundamental Movements: Focus on compound exercises like squats, lunges, push-ups, and rows.

Progression: Start with bodyweight exercises and gradually increase resistance using dumbbells, resistance bands, or weight machines.

Remember: Form is everything. Lifting heavy with poor form is a fast track to injury. Start light and focus on technique.

Cardiovascular Fitness: More Than Just a Treadmill

Cardio doesn't have to mean running on a treadmill until you're bored to tears. Find what you enjoy, whether it's cycling, swimming, hiking, or dancing.

Frequency: 3-5 days per week for at least 30 minutes.

Intensity: Mix it up! Use a combination of steady-state cardio and high-intensity interval training (HIIT) to keep your heart healthy and workouts engaging.

Flexibility and Recovery: The Secret Weapons

It's easy to overlook flexibility and recovery, but they're the unsung heroes of a balanced fitness routine. Think of them as the oil that keeps your engine running smoothly.

Daily Stretching: Spend at least 10-15 minutes stretching major muscle groups.
Recovery Tools: Foam rollers, massage guns, and yoga sessions can work wonders for post-exercise soreness.
Active Rest Days: Use rest days for light activities like walking or a gentle yoga session to keep blood flowing and prevent stiffness.

Common Mistakes to Avoid

Let's be honest: We all make mistakes. However, in fitness, some errors can lead to setbacks or even injuries.

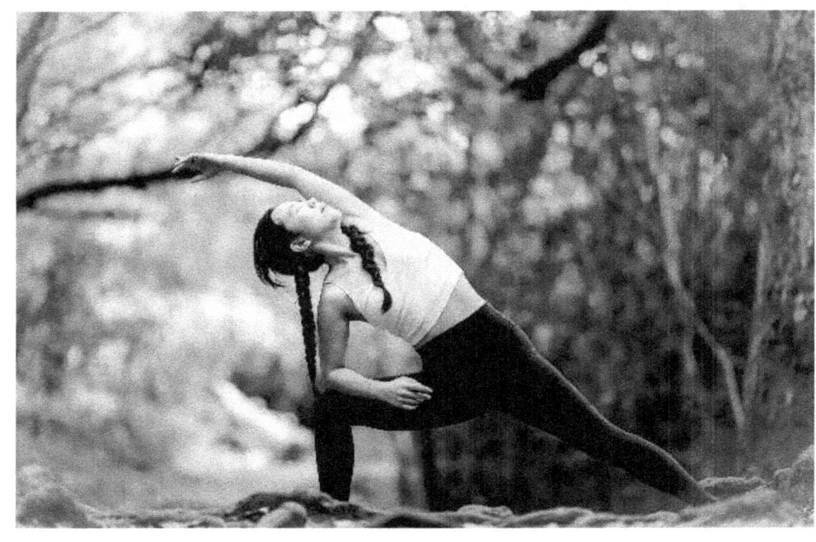

- **Overtraining:** Your body needs time to recover. Pushing too hard too often is counterproductive.
- **Skipping Warm-Ups:** A proper warm-up primes your muscles and joints, reducing the risk of injury.
- **Ignoring Flexibility:** Poor flexibility can compromise your strength and make you more injury-prone.

Tracking Your Progress

Progress isn't always measured by the number on a scale. Take note of how you feel, move, and recover. Here are a few ways to keep track:

- **Workout Journal:** Record exercises, sets, and how you felt during each session.
- **Weekly Check-Ins:** Assess your energy levels, mood, and any changes in how your clothes fit.
- **Milestone Goals:** Celebrate when you hit a milestone, whether it's lifting heavier weights or running farther.

Making Exercise a Lifestyle, Not a Chore

The goal of *Graded Exercise* is to create a sustainable routine that fits your life. It's not about punishing yourself for what you ate or chasing unrealistic goals. It's about feeling strong, capable, and full of life.

Remember: Exercise is a gift you give yourself, not a punishment. Enjoy the process, stay consistent, and your body will reward you with strength and resilience.

Chapter 5: Attitude is Everything—Mindset and Motivation

Your body follows where your mind leads. You're not alone if you're struggling with sticking to health goals or feeling motivated. Our minds can be our biggest allies or our most significant obstacles. This chapter dives into harnessing your mental strength so you can stay motivated, positive, and resilient.

The Power of a Growth Mindset

Adopting a growth mindset means seeing challenges as opportunities, not obstacles. Instead of believing your current abilities limit you, you understand that effort and perseverance lead to improvement.

Fixed vs. Growth Mindset

- *Fixed Mindset*: "I'm not athletic, so I'll never be good at exercising."
- *Growth Mindset*: "I may not be athletic yet, but I can get better with practice."

Practical Tip: Keep a journal of your health and fitness journey. Note small victories, like trying a new exercise or resisting an unhealthy snack. Reflecting on progress can reinforce a growth mindset.

Visualization Techniques

Athletes often use visualization to boost performance. By picturing success—whether it's nailing a yoga pose, lifting a heavier weight, or eating a balanced meal—you prepare your brain for achievement.

How to Visualize Effectively

1. Close your eyes and take a few deep breaths.
2. Imagine yourself completing a goal with ease.
3. Feel the emotions of success—joy, pride, and satisfaction.

Try This: Spend five minutes visualizing your workout before you start. It might sound silly, but it primes your brain for a positive experience.

Setting SMART Goals

Vague goals like "get healthier" are hard to stick to. Instead, use the SMART method to create goals that are:

- **Specific**: Define exactly what you want to achieve.
- **Measurable**: Track your progress.
- **Achievable**: Be realistic.
- **Relevant**: Make it meaningful.
- **Time-Bound**: Set a deadline.

Example: Instead of "I want to lose weight," try, "I want to lose 10 pounds in 3 months by exercising three times a week and meal prepping."

Action Step: Write down three SMART goals for your wellness journey and revisit them monthly.

Handling Setbacks with Grace

We all face setbacks. Maybe it's an injury, a holiday binge, or just a bad week. The key is how you respond. Rather than spiraling into guilt or frustration, treat setbacks as learning experiences.

Practice Self-Compassion

- Talk to yourself like you would to a friend. Would you criticize a friend for missing a workout or encourage them to try again tomorrow?
- Use setbacks as data, not failure. Analyze what went wrong and plan to prevent it in the future.

Finding Your Why

Motivation isn't one-size-fits-all. To stay driven, you need a strong personal reason for your health journey. This is your "why."

Examples of a Strong Why

- To play with your kids without getting tired.
- To live pain-free and enjoy outdoor adventures.
- To feel confident and strong in your daily life.

Exercise: Write down your "why" and place it somewhere visible—your bathroom mirror, fridge, or workout gear. Seeing it daily will keep you motivated.

Surround Yourself with Positivity

Your environment influences your behavior more than you think. Surround yourself with people who uplift and support your goals and create spaces that encourage healthy choices.

Healthy Environment Tips

- Keep nutritious snacks easily accessible.
- Join a fitness group or find a workout buddy.
- Follow motivational accounts or podcasts that inspire you.

The Role of Gratitude

Gratitude shifts your focus from what you lack to what you have. This simple practice can elevate your mood and improve your attitude toward your wellness journey.

How to Practice Gratitude

1. Write down three things you're grateful for each morning.
2. Appreciate your body for what it can do rather than criticize it for what it can't.

Example: "I'm grateful for my strong legs that carry me through each day."

Wrapping Up: Your Mind is Your Greatest Tool

Mastering your mindset is like building a solid foundation for a house. With the right attitude, even the most challenging days become manageable. Remember: motivation might waver, but a well-cultivated mindset will keep you moving forward.

Let's harness the power of your mind and set you up for a lifetime of health and happiness. You've got this!

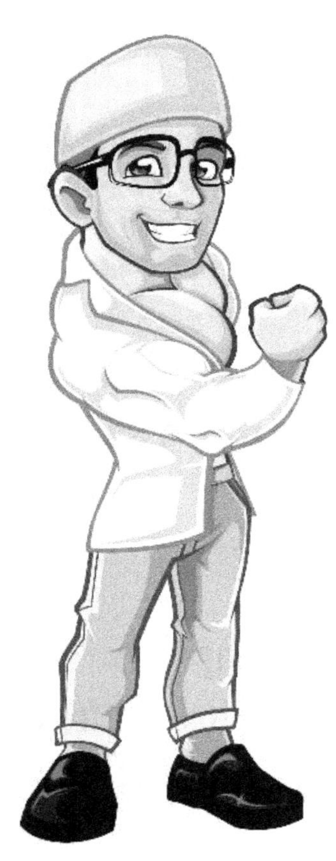

Chapter 6: Integrated Medicine—A Balanced Approach to Health

Integrated medicine isn't about choosing between modern and traditional therapies. Instead, it's about leveraging the best of all approaches to create a personalized wellness plan. This chapter explores how physician-guided strategies, targeted treatments, and alternative therapies can transform your health journey.

Physician-Guided Health Plans

Starting your journey to better health may require medical intervention, especially if you're dealing with chronic issues or metabolic dysfunction. A physician-guided approach ensures you have expert oversight, personalized recommendations, and a well-rounded plan.

Why See a Specialist First?

- **Comprehensive Assessments**: Understanding your unique health profile—whether it's hormone levels, metabolic markers, or joint stability—can guide effective interventions. This is where a specialist's expertise is crucial, as they can interpret these assessments and recommend the most suitable interventions.

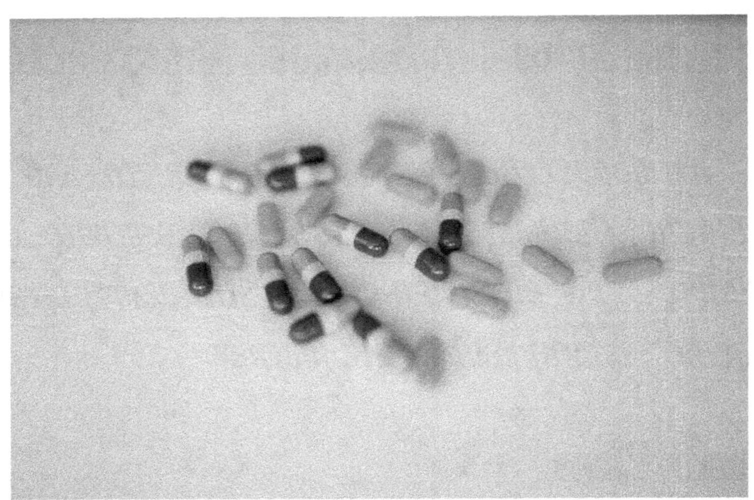

Targeted Medications: Sometimes, medications are necessary to help you get started. Let's break down a few game-changing options:

- **Metformin**: Known for its role in managing prediabetes and type 2 diabetes, metformin improves insulin sensitivity and can be an essential tool for jumpstarting metabolic health.
- **GLP-1 Receptor Agonists**: For those struggling with morbid obesity, GLP-1 medications like semaglutide have shown significant results in controlling appetite and supporting weight loss. Under the guidance of a physician, these treatments can provide the boost needed to start your health journey.
- **Contrave/Wellbutrin**: Appetite control and motivation. If you struggle with motivation and a compelling feeling to eat, this may be a medication for you and your doctor to consider. Consider the side effects and risks with your doctor.

Key Point: While these medications are powerful tools, they are part of a broader strategy that includes lifestyle and dietary changes. At Prisk Orthopaedics and Wellness, we focus on integrating these treatments into a holistic plan.

Physical Therapy Assessments and Treatments

Movement as Medicine

Physical therapy isn't just for injury recovery—it's a proactive strategy to improve mobility, prevent injuries, and enhance overall well-being. Here's how it fits into the G.A.I.N. Plan:

- **Joint Health and Stability**: Tailored exercises strengthen stabilizing muscles and improve joint function.
- **Post-Injury Rehabilitation**: Recover faster and smarter with expert-guided therapy.

Visit Us: At Prisk Orthopaedics and Wellness, our physical therapy assessments identify movement imbalances and set you on a path to pain-free activity.

Supplements That Act Like Medicine

Supplements can play a crucial role in filling gaps and supporting your body's natural healing processes. Here are some powerful options:

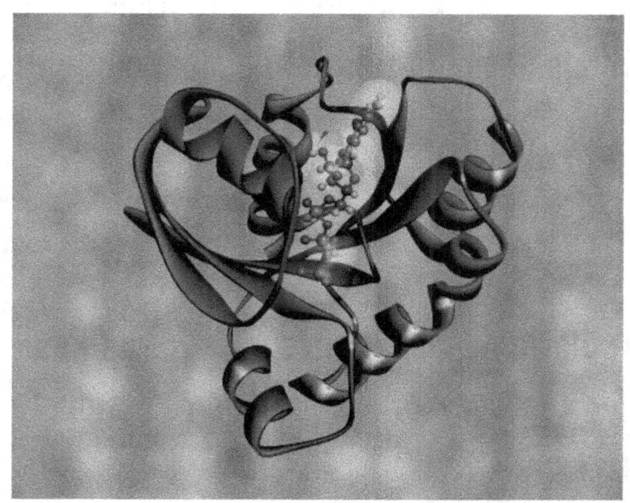

- **Leucine**: This amino acid not only boosts muscle protein synthesis but also regulates metabolism in a way similar to GLP-1 receptor agonists. It's especially beneficial during weight loss and aging.
- **Berberine**: Often compared to metformin, berberine improves insulin sensitivity and regulates blood sugar. It's a natural alternative for metabolic health, perfect for those looking to reduce their reliance on medication.
- **Fenugreek**: This herb has shown promise in lowering HbA1c levels and improving blood sugar control.
- **Ashwagandha**: An adaptogen that regulates cortisol, lowers stress, and balances hormones—crucial for both mental and physical health.

Ask About Our Supplement Guidance: We offer personalized recommendations and safe integration into your health plan.

The Role of Alternative Therapies

Incorporating therapies like massage, acupuncture, and mindfulness practices can significantly enhance your wellness plan. These methods not only relieve physical pain but also reduce stress and improve overall health.

Massage Therapy

- **Benefits**: Reduces muscle tension, improves circulation, and lowers stress hormones.
- **Applications**: Whether it's a sports massage for recovery or a relaxation session to ease stress, massage therapy can be transformative.

Acupuncture

- **How It Works**: By stimulating specific points in the body, acupuncture balances energy flow and provides pain relief.
- **Benefits**: Effective for managing pain, reducing anxiety, and improving sleep.

Mindfulness and Meditation

Practices like mindfulness and deep breathing reduce stress and improve mental clarity. These are critical components of integrated health, enhancing your overall well-being.

Explore These Therapies at Our Practice: We offer guidance on which therapies might work best for you, ensuring they complement your comprehensive health plan.

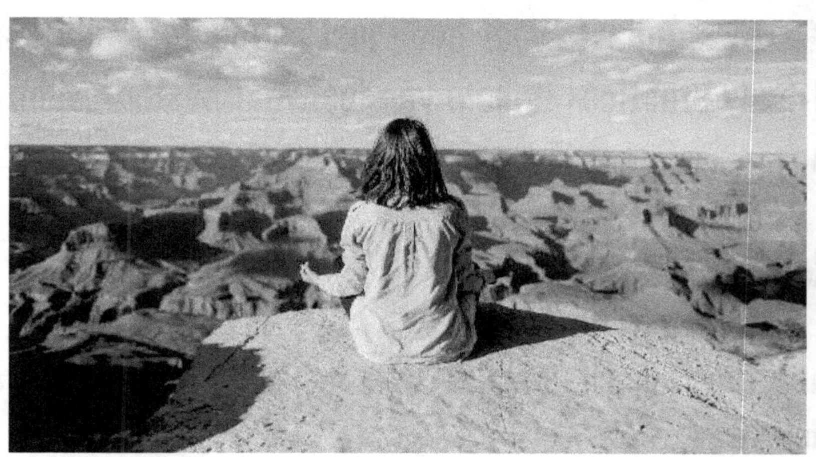

Supplements for Joint and Overall Health

Your joints work hard every day, so keeping them healthy is essential. Here are some supplements we often recommend:

- **Collagen**: Supports joint health, skin elasticity, and muscle recovery. Great for athletes and those with joint pain.
- **Omega-3 Fatty Acids**: Powerful anti-inflammatory properties that benefit heart health and reduce joint pain.
- **Magnesium**: Vital for muscle relaxation and overall wellness. Helps with sleep, stress, and muscle cramps.

Get a Customized Plan: At Prisk Orthopaedics and Wellness, we'll develop a supplement strategy tailored to your needs, ensuring safety and effectiveness.

Stress Reduction Techniques

We understand that stress impacts your body just as much as physical injury. That's why we emphasize mind-body practices to help you feel your best, providing relief and comfort in your health journey.

Effective Stress-Relievers

- **Tai Chi**: A gentle, low-impact practice that reduces inflammation and treats insomnia, making it a holistic way to stay active.
- **Yoga and Deep Breathing**: These methods lower stress hormones and improve flexibility.
- **Matcha for Oral Health**: Research shows it can inhibit bacteria that cause gum disease, adding to its reputation as a stress-relieving superfood.

Join Our Wellness Programs: We offer workshops and classes that focus on reducing stress and enhancing your overall well-being. By joining these programs, you'll become part of a supportive community that is dedicated to your health and wellness.

Bringing It All Together

Integrated medicine at Prisk Orthopaedics and Wellness means having a comprehensive, personalized plan that uses every available tool to improve your health. This approach is designed to inspire and empower you, giving you the tools and knowledge to take control of your health and achieve lasting wellness.

Ready to take control of your health? Schedule a consultation with us today and begin your journey toward optimal wellness.

NOTES

Chapter 7: The Power of Leucine and Nutrient Timing

Imagine a nutrient so powerful that it can flip a switch in your body to build muscle, burn fat, and improve your metabolic health. Leucine, an essential amino acid, holds the key to unlocking these benefits. In this chapter, we'll explore why leucine deserves your attention and how nutrient timing can amplify your results.

The Science of Leucine: More Than Just an Amino Acid

Leucine is more than just one of the building blocks of protein—it's a *master regulator* of muscle protein synthesis. In simpler terms, leucine is like the CEO of your muscle metabolism, calling the shots and ensuring your body prioritizes building and repairing muscle.

Mother's Milk: Nature's Blueprint for Growth

Let's take a moment to appreciate one of the most telling sources of leucine: *mother's milk*. In my research while writing *The G.A.I.N. Plan* and *The Leucine Factor Diet*, I highlighted that breast milk is naturally rich in leucine, which underscores the critical role this amino acid plays in growth and development. It's nature's way of ensuring that infants receive the essential nutrients needed for rapid muscle and tissue growth, setting a foundation for lifelong health.

Key Insight: If leucine is so essential for an infant's development, it stands to reason that it continues to play a crucial role in maintaining and optimizing muscle mass and metabolic health throughout adulthood.

Why Leucine is a Game-Changer for Adults

As we age, our ability to maintain muscle mass and metabolic health declines. Leucine becomes even more important for:

- **Preventing Muscle Loss (Sarcopenia)**: Muscle loss is a major health concern as we age. Leucine triggers the mTOR pathway, which is responsible for muscle protein synthesis, helping to combat sarcopenia.
- **Optimizing Metabolism**: Muscle tissue is metabolically active, meaning it burns more calories at rest. By maintaining and building muscle through adequate leucine intake, you can boost your resting metabolic rate.
- **Controlling Blood Sugar**: Leucine helps regulate insulin and supports blood sugar control, acting in ways similar to certain diabetes medications.

How Much Leucine Do You Need?

Based on my research, consuming **2.5 to 3 grams of leucine per meal** is optimal to trigger muscle protein synthesis. This is especially important for older adults, athletes, or anyone aiming to improve body composition. *SEE THE POWFIT TRAINER ONLINE @ POWFIT.COM

Leucine-Rich Foods

- **Whey Protein**: A complete protein source with high leucine content, ideal for post-workout recovery.
- **Eggs**: Nature's perfect protein, with a high biological value and a leucine boost.
- **Chicken Breast**: Lean and protein-rich, providing a substantial amount of leucine.
- **Soy Products**: For plant-based eaters, tofu and tempeh are solid options that supply leucine.

Practical Tip: Aim to distribute your leucine intake evenly across meals to maximize muscle protein synthesis throughout the day.

Leucine's Role in Fat Loss and Muscle Maintenance

In *The Leucine Factor Diet*, I emphasized that leucine is not only critical for muscle building but also for *maintaining lean muscle mass during weight loss*. Unlike typical dieting approaches that often lead to muscle loss, a leucine-focused diet preserves muscle, ensuring your metabolism stays efficient.

How Leucine Affects Fat Loss

- Leucine increases energy expenditure by supporting muscle mass.
- It also helps curb hunger by regulating satiety hormones, making it easier to adhere to a calorie-controlled diet.

Connecting Leucine to Nutrient Timing

While the concept of the anabolic window has been broadened, timing your leucine intake around workouts can still provide benefits, especially for muscle recovery and growth.

Leucine Post-Workout

- After intense exercise, your muscles are more receptive to protein synthesis. Consuming a protein source rich in leucine within a few hours post-workout maximizes recovery.
- If you're training fasted or it's been a while since your last meal, having a leucine-rich protein shake post-exercise is particularly effective.

Reinforcement: This principle connects back to the insight from mother's milk. Just as infants thrive with a constant supply of leucine-rich nutrients, adults can optimize muscle health with strategic leucine intake.

Supplements That Complement Leucine

Your approach in *The G.A.I.N. Plan* and *The Leucine Factor Diet* emphasizes a balance between natural food sources and supplementation. Here are additional supplements that enhance leucine's benefits:

- **HMB (Beta-Hydroxy Beta-Methylbutyrate)**: Derived from leucine, HMB is highly effective at reducing muscle breakdown, making it ideal for individuals on calorie-restricted diets or older adults.
- **Creatine**: Supports energy production in muscles, complementing leucine's muscle-building effects.
- **Omega-3 Fatty Acids**: These anti-inflammatory fats support muscle recovery and joint health, essential for anyone active or dealing with chronic inflammation.

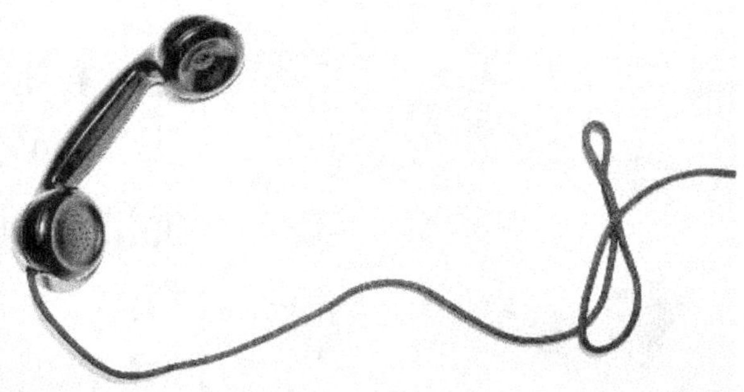

How Leucine and Other Supplements Act Like Medications

Some supplements have effects that mimic those of traditional medications, making them valuable in a comprehensive wellness plan:

- **Leucine and GLP-1**: Leucine influences insulin and blood sugar regulation similarly to GLP-1 receptor agonists, supporting metabolic health.
- **Berberine and Metformin**: Berberine is a natural compound that works much like metformin, improving insulin sensitivity and lowering blood sugar levels.
- **Fenugreek for Blood Sugar**: This herb has been shown to reduce HbA1c and improve glycemic control.
- **Ashwagandha for Stress**: This adaptogen helps balance cortisol, lowering stress and supporting recovery.

Making Nutrient Timing Work for You

Here are some practical ways to incorporate these principles into your daily routine:

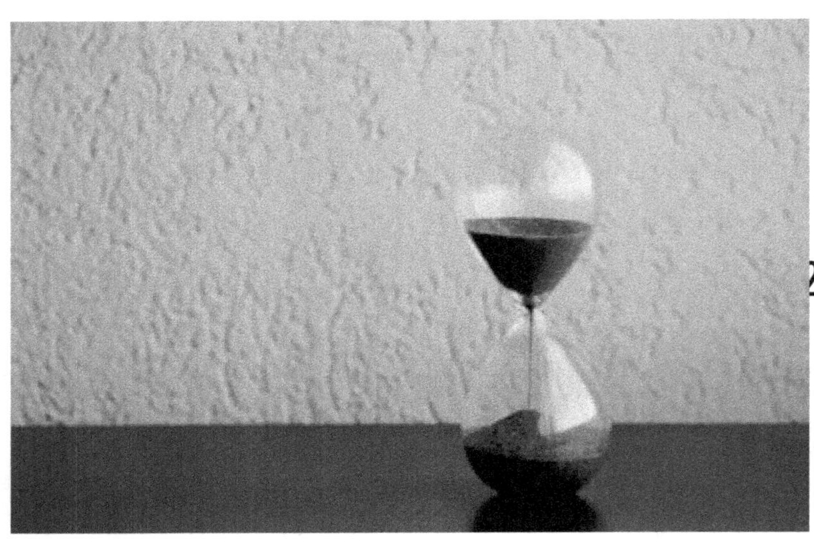

1. **Plan Your Protein**: Make sure each meal contains 20-30 grams of high-quality protein, with enough leucine to trigger muscle growth.
2. **Post-Workout Nutrition**: While the anabolic window isn't as narrow as once thought, having a protein-rich meal post-workout is still a good practice, especially if it's been several hours since your last meal.
3. **Balance is Key**: While leucine is crucial, remember that a balanced diet rich in whole foods is the foundation of good health.

Bringing It All Together

Understanding leucine and nutrient timing can transform your approach to nutrition and exercise. These principles aren't just for athletes—they're for anyone looking to improve body composition, boost metabolism, and live a healthier, more active life.

Contact Us: At Prisk Orthopaedics and Wellness, we're passionate about helping you harness the power of leucine and build a diet plan that supports your unique needs. Schedule a consultation today! 412-525-POW2

Chapter 8: Meal Planning for Health and Recovery

You've learned the science behind leucine and nutrient timing. Now, it's time to put it all into action with meal planning that fuels your body, maximizes recovery, and keeps you on track with your wellness goals. In this chapter, I'll guide you through creating balanced meals and strategies for making meal prep an essential part of your health journey.

Why Meal Planning Matters

Meal planning isn't just for fitness enthusiasts or nutrition nerds. It's a game-changer for anyone trying to live a healthier life. By planning your meals, you can ensure you're getting enough leucine, quality protein, healthy fats, and nutrient-dense carbohydrates— all while saving time and avoiding the temptation of less nutritious convenience foods.

Benefits of Meal Planning

- **Consistency**: It's easier to hit your daily protein and leucine targets when you plan ahead.
- **Portion Control**: Pre-planned meals help you manage portion sizes and avoid mindless eating.
- **Budget-Friendly**: Cooking at home is generally cheaper than dining out or ordering takeout.

The Basics of a Balanced Meal

For optimal health and recovery, every meal should be built with these key components:

1. High-Quality Protein

Protein is the star of the show. Aim for 20-30 grams per meal, with a focus on leucine-rich sources to stimulate muscle protein synthesis.

Examples:

- Grilled chicken breast (3 oz) = ~26g protein

    - Whey protein shake = ~25g protein
    - Tofu (4 oz) = ~14g protein

1. **Complex Carbohydrates**

   Carbs are your primary source of energy. Choose whole, nutrient-dense options like quinoa, brown rice, sweet potatoes, and legumes. They provide steady energy and help replenish muscle glycogen post-workout.

2. **Healthy Fats**

   Don't be afraid of fat! Healthy fats support hormone production, brain function, and joint health. Include sources like avocado, olive oil, nuts, and seeds in your meals.

3. **Colorful Vegetables**

   Vegetables add vitamins, minerals, and antioxidants to your diet. Aim to "eat the rainbow" and include a variety of veggies at each meal.

Example Balanced Meal:

- **Protein**: Grilled salmon (4 oz)
- **Carbs**: Quinoa (1 cup)
- **Fats**: Avocado slices
- **Veggies**: Roasted broccoli and bell peppers

You've already learned about nutrient timing, but let's break it down into practical steps:

Meal Timing and Distribution

1. **Breakfast**: Start your day with a protein-rich breakfast to kickstart muscle protein synthesis.

   Example: Scrambled eggs with spinach, whole-grain toast, and a side of mixed berries.

2. **Post-Workout Meal**: After a workout, focus on a meal that includes protein and carbs to optimize recovery.

   Example: Whey protein shake blended with a banana and almond milk.

3. **Evening Meals**: A well-rounded dinner helps repair muscles and keeps you satiated.

   Example: Baked chicken with roasted sweet potatoes and a leafy green salad.

Practical Tip: Spacing your protein evenly throughout the day, rather than loading it all into one meal, helps maintain muscle protein synthesis.

Meal Prep Strategies for Success

1. Batch Cooking

Dedicate a day each week to cook and portion out meals. This way, you always have healthy options ready to go, and it minimizes the temptation to reach for less nutritious choices.

2. Use a Slow Cooker or Instant Pot

These appliances are perfect for cooking large quantities of protein, like shredded chicken or beef stew, with minimal effort.

3. Invest in Quality Containers

Reusable glass containers keep your meals fresh and make portioning easier. Plus, they're microwave-safe for quick reheating.

Leucine-Focused Meal Ideas

Here are some meal and snack ideas to help you hit your leucine targets:

Breakfast

- **Leucine-Packed Smoothie**: Blend whey protein, spinach, frozen berries, almond milk, and a tablespoon of chia seeds.
- **Greek Yogurt Bowl**: Top Greek yogurt with sliced almonds, chia seeds, and a drizzle of honey.

Lunch

- **Power Bowl**: Quinoa base topped with grilled chicken, black beans, diced avocado, and roasted vegetables.
- **High-Protein Salad**: Spinach, grilled salmon, boiled eggs, cherry tomatoes, and a tahini dressing.

Dinner

- **Leucine-Loaded Stir Fry**: Lean beef or tofu with mixed vegetables, served over brown rice or cauliflower rice.
- **Baked Cod and Sweet Potatoes**: Serve with a side of sautéed kale and garlic.

Snacks

- **Edamame**: A great plant-based source of leucine.
- **Cottage Cheese and Pineapple**: A high-protein snack with a touch of natural sweetness.
- **Protein Bars**: Choose ones with high leucine content and minimal added sugars.

Supplements for Meal Planning

While whole foods should make up the bulk of your nutrition, supplements can fill in the gaps:

- **Whey Protein**: Convenient for post-workout nutrition or when you need a quick leucine boost.
- **Casein Protein**: A slow-digesting protein, great for a nighttime shake to support muscle recovery.
- **BCAAs**: If you're in a calorie deficit or need an intra-workout boost, branched-chain amino acids (including leucine) can be beneficial.

Eating Out: Making Smart Choices

Dining out doesn't have to derail your progress. Here's how to keep it healthy:

1. **Choose Lean Proteins**: Opt for grilled, baked, or broiled options instead of fried.
2. **Swap Sides**: Replace fries or white rice with a side salad or steamed vegetables.
3. **Watch the Sauces**: Dressings and sauces often contain hidden sugars and fats. Ask for them on the side.

Example Dining Out Meal: A balanced and nutritious meal, such as grilled salmon with a side of roasted vegetables and a mixed greens salad, can provide a good source of protein, healthy fats, and a variety of vitamins and minerals.

Your Personalized Meal Plan

Creating a meal plan tailored to your needs can make all the difference in achieving your health goals. Remember, it's not about perfection but consistency. Aim to nourish your body, hit your leucine targets, and enjoy the process.

Chapter 9: Sustaining Progress and Adjusting Goals

Making lasting changes to your health and fitness isn't a sprint; it's a marathon. You've learned the principles of the G.A.I.N. Plan and the science behind leucine, nutrition, and exercise. Now it's time to talk about sustaining your progress, adjusting your goals as needed, and staying motivated for the long haul.

The Importance of Progress Tracking

Tracking your progress keeps you accountable and helps you recognize the small victories that add up to significant changes over time. But what should you be tracking, and how?

1. Physical Measurements

- **Weight and Body Composition**: Use a scale, but don't get too caught up in daily fluctuations. If possible, measure your body fat percentage and muscle mass using a reliable method, like a DEXA scan or body composition analyzer.
- **Circumference Measurements**: Track your waist, hips, thighs, arms, and chest to see where you're losing fat or gaining muscle.
- **Photos**: Progress photos are a great way to track your changes over weeks and months visually.

2. Performance Metrics

- **Strength Gains**: Log the weights you lift and the number of reps and sets you complete. If you're lifting more or performing more reps over time, you're making progress.
- **Endurance**: Track how far or how long you can run, cycle, or swim. Improvements in stamina are clear signs of cardiovascular progress.
- **Flexibility**: Note how your range of motion improves, especially if you've been working on mobility exercises.

3. Health Markers

- **Blood Pressure and Heart Rate**: These can indicate improvements in cardiovascular health.
- **Blood Work**: Keep an eye on cholesterol, HbA1c, and inflammatory markers. Your doctor can help you interpret these results.

Practical Tip: Use a journal or an app to track these metrics. Seeing your progress laid out can be incredibly motivating.

Adjusting Your Goals

As you make progress, your goals will naturally evolve. Here's how to adjust them effectively:

1. Reassess Your "Why"

The reasons you started your wellness journey may change over time. Perhaps you initially wanted to lose weight, but now your focus has shifted to building strength or running a marathon. Reconnect with your core motivations and adjust your goals accordingly.

2. Set New SMART Goals

Remember the SMART framework: Specific, Measurable, Achievable, Relevant, and Time-Bound. This means your goals should be clear and specific, you should be able to measure your progress, they should be realistic and relevant to your overall health and fitness, and they should have a deadline for completion. As you reach your initial targets, create new ones to keep the momentum going.

Example: If your first goal was to lose 10 pounds, your next might be to run a 5K race in under 30 minutes or bench press your body weight.

3. Celebrate Your Achievements

Don't forget to celebrate your victories, both big and small. Whether it's treating yourself to a massage, buying new workout gear, or taking a day off to relax, rewards can reinforce positive behavior.

Remember: Progress isn't always linear. There will be plateaus and setbacks, but the key is to stay adaptable and keep moving forward. Two steps forward, one step back is still moving forward.

Staying Motivated: Tips for the Long Haul

Motivation can be fleeting, but discipline and smart strategies will carry you through even when your enthusiasm wanes. Here are some practical ways to stay motivated:

1. Mix Up Your Routine

Boredom is a motivation killer. Keep your workouts exciting by trying new activities, like kickboxing, rock climbing, or paddleboarding. In the gym, change up your exercises every few weeks to keep your muscles guessing.

2. Join a Community

Having a support system can make all the difference. Whether it's a gym class, a running club, or an online fitness group, being part of a community adds accountability and makes fitness more fun.

3. Use Visualization Techniques

Visualizing your success can keep you focused on your goals. Picture yourself crossing the finish line of that race or lifting a new personal best. This mental exercise can boost your confidence and motivation.

4. Keep a Gratitude Journal

It's easy to get fixated on what you haven't achieved yet. A gratitude journal can shift your focus to the positive. Write down three things you're grateful for each day, whether it's your improving health, supportive friends, or the strength to complete a tough workout.

When to Seek Professional Guidance

Sometimes, despite your best efforts, you might feel stuck. That's when it's time to bring in the experts. Here's how our team at Prisk Orthopaedics and Wellness can help:

- **Nutrition Counseling**: If you're struggling with meal planning or hitting a plateau, a nutritionist can offer personalized advice to get you back on track.
- **Physical Therapy**: Experiencing nagging pain or discomfort? A physical therapist can assess your movement patterns and create a plan to prevent injury.
- **Strength and Conditioning Coaching**: A personal trainer can help you fine-tune your workouts and ensure you're using proper form.

The Power of Reflection

Take time to reflect on how far you've come. Remember when even a short walk felt like a chore? Or when meal prepping seemed overwhelming? Reflecting on your progress can give you a newfound appreciation for your efforts and the resilience you've developed.

Questions to Ponder

1. What have I learned about myself since starting this journey?
2. How has my relationship with food and exercise evolved?
3. What are the habits I've developed that I'm most proud of?

Looking Forward

The journey to optimal health is ongoing. There's always room for growth, new goals to achieve, and new challenges to tackle. Stay curious, keep learning, and remember that every step forward, no matter how small, is progress.

NOTES

Chapter 10: Real-Life Success Stories and Practical Tips

Sometimes, what we need most is proof that lasting change is possible. Throughout my career, I've witnessed incredible transformations—stories that remind us of the power of perseverance, discipline, and a well-structured plan. In this chapter, we'll explore some real-life success stories and extract the practical lessons that can apply to your own journey.

The Power of Transformation: Real-Life Stories

Let's start with a few inspiring stories from my patients and clients who embraced the G.A.I.N. principles and changed their lives.

What Worked for Maria:

Maria's Journey: From Chronic Pain to Running Again

Maria, 45, came to me with chronic knee pain. Years of discomfort had taken a toll on her both physically and mentally, and she had all but given up on being active. But through a combination of physician-guided physical therapy, strength training, and a leucine-rich diet, Maria made incredible progress.

- **Graded Exercise**: We started with low-impact exercises that strengthened her knee and improved her overall mobility. As she got stronger, we gradually introduced more challenging activities.
- **Nutrition**: Maria incorporated high-leucine foods, which helped her maintain muscle mass while reducing inflammation.
- **Mindset Shift**: Visualization exercises helped Maria regain confidence in her body. She could finally picture herself pain-free and active.

Outcome: Within eight months, Maria was jogging pain-free and had completed her first 5K race. She says she feels stronger than she has in years.

David's Story: Reversing Metabolic Syndrome

David, 52, was diagnosed with metabolic syndrome—high blood pressure, high blood sugar, and excess body fat around his waist. He needed to make drastic changes to avoid a lifetime of medication. We worked together to create a comprehensive plan using the G.A.I.N. principles.

What Worked for David:

- **Integrated Medicine**: Initially, David was prescribed metformin to help regulate his blood sugar. However, we complemented this with a structured diet plan rich in leucine and whole foods.
- **Exercise Routine**: We focused on weight training and cardio, gradually increasing the intensity as his body adapted.
- **Stress Management**: David started practicing mindfulness and deep breathing exercises, which helped lower his blood pressure and reduce stress.

Outcome: Over the course of a year, David lost 35 pounds, reduced his waist circumference by six inches, and was able to discontinue metformin under his physician's guidance. His blood pressure and blood sugar levels normalized, and he felt more energetic than ever.

Sarah's Triumph: Beating Burnout and Finding Strength

Sarah, 38, was a busy executive who suffered from chronic fatigue and felt overwhelmed by stress. Her work-life balance was non-existent, and her health was suffering as a result. We developed a holistic wellness plan that fits into her demanding schedule.

What Worked for Sarah:

- **Graded Exercise**: Short, high-intensity interval training (HIIT) workouts allowed Sarah to stay fit despite her busy schedule.
- **Adaptogens**: We introduced ashwagandha and magnesium supplements to help manage her stress and improve sleep quality.
- **Leucine and Nutrition**: Meal prepping with high-leucine foods helped Sarah stay energized and avoid the afternoon crash.

Outcome: Within six months, Sarah reported feeling more energetic, sleeping better, and even excelling at work, thanks to improved mental clarity and focus. She found a passion for yoga, which became her go-to stress relief activity.

Lesson: Small, strategic changes can lead to big improvements, even for the busiest individuals.

Practical Tips for Everyday Life

Drawing from these success stories, here are practical tips that you can implement in your own journey:

1. Make Health Non-Negotiable

Treat your health like an essential meeting that you cannot skip. Schedule your workouts and meal prep sessions like you would any other important commitment.

2. Keep It Simple

You don't need an elaborate plan to get started. Focus on making small, manageable changes, like walking for 20 minutes a day or adding an extra serving of vegetables to your meals.

3. Find Activities You Enjoy

If you hate running, don't force yourself to do it. There are countless ways to stay active— find something that you genuinely look forward to, like swimming, dancing, or hiking.

4. Prioritize Recovery

Your muscles grow and repair during rest, not during exercise. Make sure you're getting adequate sleep and incorporating rest days into your routine.

5. Use Visual Cues

Keep your running shoes by the door, have a water bottle on your desk, or set reminders on your phone to stand and stretch. These cues can serve as gentle reminders to stay on track.

Your Journey is Unique

Everyone's path to wellness looks different. It's not about comparing your progress to someone else's but staying focused on your own goals and improvements. Remember, even the smallest victories deserve to be celebrated.

Join Us: At Prisk Orthopaedics and Wellness, we celebrate every step of your journey. If you're ready to take your health to the next level, schedule a consultation with us. Together, we can achieve amazing things.

Conclusion: Your Journey to Health and Wellness

Congratulations on making it to the end of this book! But let's be honest: this isn't the end of your wellness journey; it's just the beginning. By embracing the principles of the G.A.I.N. Plan and understanding the power of leucine, nutrient timing, and integrated medicine, you are now equipped with the knowledge to transform your health. The real question is: What will you do with this newfound knowledge?

Reflecting on Your Progress

Take a moment to reflect on everything you've learned. From the importance of balanced nutrition to the critical role of mindset, you now have a comprehensive toolkit to make lasting changes. Remember, transformation doesn't happen overnight. It's a series of small, consistent steps that lead to monumental progress.

Recap of Key Takeaways:

1. **Graded Exercise**: Start where you are and build progressively. Your body will thank you for taking a measured approach rather than diving into extreme routines.
2. **Attitude**: A positive, resilient mindset can change everything. Visualize your success and stay focused on your "why."
3. **Integrated Medicine**: A balanced approach to wellness means leveraging modern medicine when needed but always prioritizing lifestyle changes for long-term success.
4. **Nutrition and Leucine**: Prioritize leucine-rich foods and focus on nutrient timing to optimize muscle growth, metabolic health, and overall wellness.

The G.A.I.N. Philosophy for Lifelong Health

The G.A.I.N. Plan isn't just a set of rules; it's a way of living. Whether you're recovering from an injury, looking to improve your fitness, or simply aiming to live a more vibrant, active life, these principles can guide you. Keep coming back to the core tenets of graded exercise, attitude, integrated medicine, and nutrition whenever you feel off track.

Remember: Wellness is not about perfection. It's about making better choices, one day at a time, and always striving to do what's best for your body and mind.

Staying Inspired and Informed

The world of health and wellness is always evolving. New research, techniques, and insights will continue to emerge. Stay curious and keep learning. Surround yourself with people who inspire and support you, and don't hesitate to reach out for help when you need it.

Our Commitment to You:

At Prisk Orthopaedics and Wellness, we are here to support you every step of the way. Whether you need guidance on nutrition, help with injury recovery, or a customized wellness plan, our team is dedicated to helping you reach your goals.

Your health is your most valuable asset. Invest in it, nurture it, and watch how it transforms every aspect of your life.

A Final Call to Action

So, what's next? Take a moment to write down your immediat scheduling a workout, planning a protein-rich meal, or booki specialist. Whatever it is, take action today. Small steps add u your best.

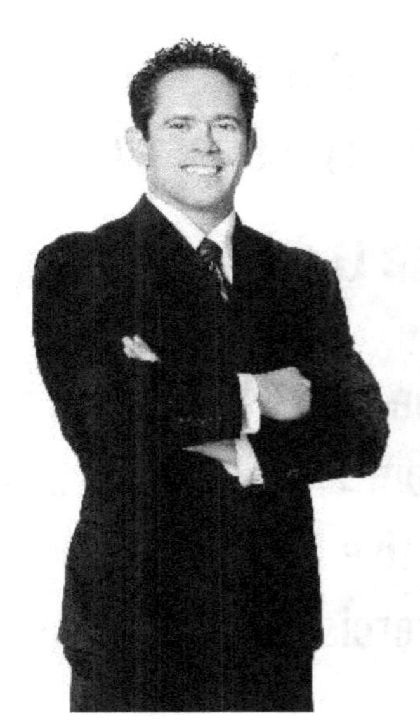

Thank You for Trusting Me

I'm honored to have shared this journey with you. Writing *The G.A.I.N. Plan* and *The Leucine Factor Diet* has been a labor of love, and I'm thrilled to see these principles come to life for readers like you. Remember, you have the power to transform your health, and I'm here to cheer you on.

Let's keep growing, learning, and thriving—together. Your best self is waiting, and it's time to G.A.I.N. your life back.

With gratitude and commitment,

www.ingramcontent.com/pod-product-compliance
Lightning Source LLC
Chambersburg PA
CBHW081811250726
48653CB00010B/3884